FATIGUE
A STEP-BY-STEP GUIDE ON HOW TO OVERCOME CHRONIC FATIGUE AND ADRENAL FATIGUE IN 30 DAYS

Sabrina Wondraczek

Published in Germany by:

Stefan Corsten
Mürrigerstr. 9
41068 Mönchengladbach

© Copyright 2015

This document is geared towards providing exact and reliable information in regards to the topic and issue covered. The publication is sold with the idea that the publisher is not required to render accounting, officially permitted, or otherwise, qualified services. If advice is necessary, legal or professional, a practiced individual in the profession should be ordered.

- From a Declaration of Principles which was accepted and approved equally by a Committee of the American Bar Association and a Committee of Publishers and Associations.

The information herein is offered for informational purposes solely, and is universal as so. The presentation of the information is without contract or any type of guarantee assurance.

Index

Introduction

I want to thank you and congratulate you for downloading the book, "Fatigue – A step-by-step Guide on how to overcome Chronic Fatigue and Adrenal Fatigue in 30 days".

This book has actionable steps and strategies on how to get rid of chronic fatigue and claim back your energy.

It is very interesting how we always seem to be in a hurry. From eating too fast, rushing from one place to another, not sleeping enough so that we can get the children ready to school or finish some assignment, working fast to meet deadlines etc; we have too much to do yet we feel we have too little time to do all there is to do. This constant frenzy makes us not have time to rest and reenergize our body to handle the daily activities. You need to understand that as human beings, we are like batteries so when we have no energy, we cannot function, as we should. This is what chronic fatigue is all about.

This book will help you understand chronic

fatigue, its causes, as well as symptoms. You will also learn how to follow a 4-week program to put an end to chronic fatigue. Simply embrace the strategies outlined in this book for only one month and trust me, your energy levels will have increased. You would wonder why you had not done what you did before!

Thanks again for downloading this book, I hope you enjoy it!

Background Information on Chronic Fatigue

It is a fact that we all feel tired from time to time. However, if you consistently experience lack of energy to perform your day-to-day obligations and feel unmotivated, then you might be suffering from chronic fatigue.

Chronic fatigue is usually an indication that there is a problem with your mitochondrial functioning among other failed body functions. It's important to know that fatigue is only a symptom of an underlying problem in your body mechanism and not a disease.

It is characterized by hormonal imbalance, toxic overload, nutrient imbalance, inadequate sleep, stress, immune dysfunction, genetic predispositions, and chronic infections.

Some common symptoms of chronic fatigue include; feeling mysteriously and severely tired all the time, un-refreshing sleep, pains, aches, short-term memory loss, severe concentration problems, headaches, lack of pleasure from your previous fun activities, anger, and depression.

The problem with medical treatment of chronic fatigue is that medical treatment of fatigue mostly focuses on eliminating the symptoms of fatigue and not the root cause. This means that the treatment only provides a temporary solution unlike the more natural means of eliminating fatigue from your body like diet and lifestyle changes.

So, what has lifestyle got to do with chronic fatigue? Well, according to research, the modern lifestyle of eating highly processed food, not exercising and exposure to toxins makes your body to breakdown, which means that our lifestyle is a major contributor to chronic fatigue. The good news is that the debilitating effects of full-blown fatigue can be reversed by making simple diet and lifestyle changes.

For you to put an end to your chronic fatigue problem, you will need to have a plan on how to actually make this work. I will take you through the month long program on how to end chronic fatigue.

NOTE: Although I will repeat this over and over again in the rest of the book, it is important to note that many of the things you will be doing for each particular week ought to be implemented throughout the program.

For instance, don't stop following the diet instructions that the book has suggested in week one just because you are now in week 3. Also, it doesn't mean you cannot meditate in week one. Everything ought to be somehow inculcated in your life.

But this doesn't mean you should do everything all at once otherwise it will result to a burn out. Introduce each week's regime with ease to ensure you don't end up feeling frustrated with the program.

And as you get started, you should ensure to have a journal where you can write whatever effects you notice, what you eat and what it is you do each day and each week.

This is because it can help you to spot any patterns of things you should watch out for during the program. Let's get started with the 30 day journey towards ending chronic fatigue.

We will start from the beginning and this is week 1.

Week 1: Eat and Balance Your Engery Level

In this first week, we will work towards changing your diet. But before I can reveal what it is you should eat and not eat during the first week, it is important to explain why you should and should not do things in a certain way in order to manage your chronic fatigue.

Additionally, we will discuss some other things you can do during the first week to help you overcome chronic fatigue in stages without having to exert too much pressure on yourself.

Work On Your Diet

As earlier intimated, research indicates that the modern diet is the main root cause of chronic fatigue and many other conditions in your body. If you are constantly feeding your system all the wrong foods like highly processed foods, foods high in sugars, and foods high in unhealthy fats, you are only making your body a broken down 'vessel'. Eventually, your body will begin to experience chronic fatigue among many other negative consequences. You need to remember that what you ingest can eventually upset your body's overall balance.

We all know that we need to eat a balanced diet comprising of carbohydrates, proteins, fats, fruits and vegetables for a healthy body. However, do you know what kinds of carbohydrates, for instance, you need to eat more as well as the kind of proteins and fats to eat? While eating a balanced diet is commendable, the composition of that balanced diet is most important. So, what is it you should eat?

(a) What Carbohydrates To Eat

A common cause of fatigue is the general imbalance in the consumption of foods containing carbohydrates. Therefore, your knowledge on the effects of the various types of carbohydrates can contribute a lot on your endeavor to end fatigue. You need to eat more of complex carbohydrates as well as low glycemic carbs to avoid crashes.

Glycemic index is simply a number associated with a certain kind of food that indicates the effect of the food on your glucose level. If you want constant energy levels throughout the day, you need to take foods that don't give you an energy rush and within a short time you are already experiencing a sudden dip in your blood glucose levels.

Complex carbs are processed slowly, which means that they don't cause a sudden sugar rush like low glycemic carbs.

Complex carbohydrates are also high in dietary fiber content, which helps you feel full for longer. This means that you are unlikely to overeat throughout the day since this can lead to weight gain, sluggishness, and fatigue. Fiber is also crucial for healthy digestion. For example, soluble fiber feeds the beneficial bacteria in your digestive tract, which prevents constipation, which is energy-draining.

Some examples of complex carbohydrates as well as carbohydrates with a low glycemic index includes whole grains such as buckwheat, barley, oats, brown rice, wild rice, wholegrain products like bread and pastas among others. Avoid wheat if you are allergic to gluten, as it can make your chronic fatigue worse.

(b) What Proteins To Eat

Protein contains the body building block (amino acids) and provides energy for your body. Different types of protein contain different amino acids that perform varying functions in your body.

For you to get regular, balanced, and sufficient amount of energy from proteins, ensure you include protein foods during your breakfast and lunch meals. Avoid eating foods containing lots of protein later in the day, since protein takes quite some time to be digested so you don't want to go to bed when some protein is still being digested as this can make you feel tired.

Opt for organic animal protein, such as fish, lean meat like skinned chicken and grass-fed beef, indigenous eggs, and cheese. Legumes like lentils, soybeans, garbanzo beans, kidney beans, split peas, navy beans and others are amazing sources of protein.

(c) What Fats To Eat

Healthy unsaturated fats boost your energy and alertness. Some foods containing unsaturated fats include non-dairy milk such as almond milk, avocados, grass-fed lean beef, Greek yoghurt, cottage cheese, boiled eggs, unsalted nuts and seeds, wild fish such as salmon, herring, cod, sardines, pike, sole, perch, flounder, mackerel, halibut, and Pollock. Fish and nuts contain the most essential fatty acid called omega 3 which lower the glycemic index in food.

Ensure you use oils such as canola, olive oil, macadamia nut oil, grape seed, almond, and avocado oil in place of processed vegetable oils for cooking.

Avoid most saturated fats except for coconut, which are found in dairy products such as butter, cream, and whole milk. Additionally, avoid trans fats found in French fries, doughnuts, margarines and in other processed foods. You do not need these fats at all. Read your ingredients labels carefully to ensure you avoid them.

With every meal, eat essential fats in small amounts to stabilize your energy level and enhance your digestion. Towards the end of your day, avoid eating large amount of fat to avoid digestive stress.

(d) What Fruits and Vegetables To Eat

Consume fibrous veggies such as rutabagas and celery roots, artichokes, asparagus, cucumber, pumpkin, broccoli, cabbage, scallions, leeks, eggplant, Brussels sprouts, dark leafy greens, carrots, sprouts, tomatoes, cauliflower, and squash. Fruits such as pears and raspberries are great fiber sources. To cleanse your system from toxic waste, eat fruits and vegetables, which are in season because they are naturally ripened. Visit farmers' markets to get more fresh food supplies.

NOTE: One of the best dieting strategies you can follow to put an end to chronic fatigue syndrome is to follow the exclusion or elimination diet. In the elimination diet, you should remove foods that you suspect trigger or heighten chronic fatigue to help you to determine if the symptoms improve.

On the other hand, if you are following the exclusion diet, you simply have to eliminate all foods and revert to the very basic diet for some time then start reintroducing foods later on (ensure to include one at a time) until you can now identify the specific food that triggers the symptoms. It is worth noting that these two diets might entail removing essential nutrients from your diet so it is best to do so under supervision from a doctor.

You should also identify food sensitivities by keeping a diary of what it is you eat and any symptoms you have when you eat different foods. This can be very helpful in spotting any patterns.

(e) Other Dietary Changes You Should Make

Drink enough Water

Integrate water intake into your daily diet to hydrate your body. Take 8 glasses of water daily in intervals well spread throughout your day to avoid dehydration which can wear your body down. Add a squeeze of lemon for taste and to alkalize it if you desire. If you are taking sufficient amount of water, your urine should be straw colored or pale yellow, darker urine signals dehydration and the need to take more water.

Avoid cigarette smoking

Cigarette contains harmful substances that interfere with mineral absorption while carbon monoxide in the smoke reduces blood oxygen circulation hence interferes with glucose metabolism. That is why smokers experience lower energy levels than non-smokers do.

Avoid or reduce consumption of alcohol

Alcohol burdens your liver detoxification process, dehydrates your body, interferes with sleep, and is treated as a high glycemic carb, which can exhaust most of your energy. To stabilize your energy, cut back on alcohol, take healthy fruit and vegetable juices that are more energy sustaining instead. Also, avoid other stimulating or sedating drugs such as marijuana or opiates, as they interfere with mineral absorption in your body causing fatigue.

To put all the above into perspective, we will break this up into each of the constituent meals to help you deal with chronic fatigue. To get started, we will start with the breakfast:

(f) Breakfast

Your immune system is greatly determined by the type of foods that you are taking. With a condition like chronic fatigue syndrome, you must be extra careful when it comes to watching what you eat. So, what exactly is it you should eat for breakfast?

(g) Beverages

The first thing that you should do is to put down the coffee you normally take. I know it smells good and it's hard to resist but coffee is not good for your health because it adds toxins in your body. Additionally, stimulants like coffee and other caffeinated beverages can disrupt your metabolism causing chronic fatigue. Usually, coffee provides a temporary energy boost, which wears off after a few hours leaving you more tired than you were in the first place.

The good news is that you have other healthy substitutes, which will help you improve your health such as dandelion chai, chamomile tea, and green tea. These substitutes will keep your energy levels up.

If you love drinking milk in the morning, it is perhaps necessary to know that some people have noted that taking milk heightens the symptoms that come with chronic fatigue. If you have to take milk, then go for rice milk or almond milk, which provides you with more beneficial protein than cow milk.

Additionally, please note that sugar suppresses the immune system, stimulates yeast overgrowth in the intestines, and increases inflammation. All this results to hypoglycemia, which has been linked to fatigue, sugar cravings, and anxiety. Also, don't take artificial sweeteners that contain sweetener aspartame and MSG since these have been shown to have negative effects on CFS patients.

Let's now look at the specifics on what to eat for your breakfast during the first week:

You should start by preparing a *green smoothie*

as your first task for the day. Then after a few minutes of relaxing, you can start working on your breakfast. Chamomile tea or whey protein powder drink is an ideal beverage, which you can take with brown bread and an egg cooked using olive oil. Ensure to use cold pressed nut and seed oils like hemp, linseed, grapeseed, sesame, olive oil, and sunflower oil. You can also take some oats and oatcakes for breakfast.

You can as well prepare salads that include mushrooms, bamboo shoots, cress, onion, peppers, celery, tomato, avocado, cucumber, and lettuce; feel free to add French dressing that has vinegar, mustard, lemon juice, garlic, olive oil etc. Take nuts like walnut, pistachio, hazel, Brazil, peanuts, tahini (sesame seed spread), and nut butter spreads. Try taking more of pulses since these are rich in vegetable fiber and starches.

Another great breakfast idea is to take seeds and greens; these will keep you full for longer. You can as well take bacon, fried tomatoes, smoked wild caught fish (kippers, mackerel, cod, salmon, haddock etc-ensure to watch out for smoked fish with dyes since these are not good). If you opt for tinned fish, insist on one packed in olive oil. You can also try mussels, tinned shrimps, cockles, prawns etc. You are also free to take brown rice kedgeree, homemade muesli (nuts, seeds, millet flakes and oat soaked overnight), rice porridge and rice cakes.

Ensure to avoid most fruit as this is often high in fructose, which is fermented in your body pretty fast. As such, this might interfere with the way the liver functions to correct low blood sugar making the problem even worse.

Many of the processed foods have additives; such things like sausage for instance contain rusk. You should avoid such things like grains (including wheat and rye and everything made using wheat/rye as an ingredient), alcohol, tap water, sugar, dairy products (including dried milk, yogurt, cheese, butter, and milk) and different grains such as millet, rice and corn. Additionally, you should ensure to avoid medicines/drugs that are high in corn, colorings, and lactose.

(h) Lunch

Your lunches should incorporate such things like homemade soup comprising vegetables, fish, red meat, or chicken. This should ideally be served with leftover casserole, baked potato that has been filled with homemade chili, tuna, prawns etc.

Your lunches could also include such things like cold meat, smoked fish, salami, prawns, fish (this is essentially tinned fish in olive), rusk free sausage i.e. 100% meat, and avocado.

You can as well take green vegetables with seed oils and nut oils. And if you want to, it would be great to take some salad that has lettuce, celery, tomato, peppers, cucumber etc) served with French dressing.

You can also try taking nuts and seeds served with soya yogurt. Another nice lunch idea is taking oatcakes. Feel free to take soup or salad with vegetable sticks and humus for lunch.

(i) Supper

As a rule of thumb, you should eat breakfast like an Emperor, lunch as if you are a king and take dinner as a pauper. This simply means your dinner should be light. You can take vegetables, fish, poultry, or meat. For instance, you can take chickpea/meat/vegetable stir fry served with brown rice pasta or just rice and some homemade sauce.

Your supper could also be a cooked plant based meal with some large green salad.

You can also take a supper that is rich in eggs, fish, or meat served with vegetables. Another idea is taking soya yogurt and berries, or nuts and seeds.

(j) Snacks

Limit your intake of high carbohydrate snacks like those made using white flour or white rice. You can take snacks like green smoothies or something else in those lines. But this doesn't mean that you MUST take snacks; you can avoid them if you want to.

Note: The anti-candida diet has been noted to have very positive effects towards fighting chronic fatigue syndrome. As such, you should ensure to cut down on table sugar (sucrose), yeast consumption, fructose (fruits), milk (lactose) and refined grains. Also, limit your intake of fermented products like soya sauce, vinegar, alcohol etc, stimulants like cola, coffee, tea, moulds like peanuts, mushrooms and cheese etc.

While on this kind of a diet (anti-candida diet), you should ideally take: whole grains, fish, organic white meat, fresh veggies, beans and pulses, natural yogurt, cold pressed vegetable oils for dressings, natural yogurt unless you are dairy intolerant, seeds and freshly cracked nuts etc.

Follow all the ideas we've learnt so far to master what it is you should be taking for the rest of the month-we will not repeat the diet part again in the book.

Get Physical

Activity management is a process where you set your daily goals and write down the number of health beneficial activities that you are planning to participate on that particular week. They say when you don't plan then you are automatically planning to fail and that's why this process is very important. You should have a diary where you can write and record your current activities and the amount of rest time that you are taking in order to gauge your activities and progress. This book comes in handy as the day goes by, but at this stage, the only thing that you should write down are your goals.

You should keep in mind that this is a treatment program so you should be disciplined and follow it to the latter. You can gradually increase your activities as you move forward.

Graded Exercise Therapy

After taking some time to rest and given time for food to digest, you can engage yourself with this type of exercise therapy. Graded exercise therapy is a physical activity that has a slow start and increases gradually over time. It involves activities such as stretching, range-of-motion contractions, and lastly extensions. Five minutes of this activity everyday is an effective way to start for those people who have been inactive.

As you begin this program, it is important for you to know that you are not supposed to push yourself to do the exercises to the extreme; you should instead learn how to balance the physical exercise with resting.

This therapy works on the mentality that too much exercise is not helpful to your health. So when doing this exercise, you should first try to gauge how long you can take before you start getting tired because you should avoid exercising after you feel ill or tired. If you take five minutes to get tired then your exercise time will be five minutes every day and for those who love counting in rounds they should also gauge themselves and see how many rounds is fit them.

Graded exercise therapy can help you to improve and get well more quickly. It is important to make this process a daily routine in order to make your body more active. The main goal of these therapy is to avoid activating CFS syndrome, prevent tiredness and lastly to increase the level of a patients fitness. You should make sure that you do this daily in a period of one week.

You should try to increase your frequency of physical activity to help you to perform your day-to-day activities. Exercising releases feel good hormones and we know when you start feeling good, you are likely to be less fatigued.

Make sure you choose a comfortable exercise and avoid pushing yourself too hard to avoid suffering from exercises related fatigue. If you are currently inactive, you can begin with exercising 2-3 days per week for 15-20 minutes each and increase with time.

(k) Exercises To Do During The First Week

Perform low impact aerobic exercises to enhance production of endorphins, which increase blood oxygen levels and boost your energy. Just like for everyone else, stretching and strengthening exercises are good exercises that enhance blood flow and relax muscle tension. You can start with 5 minutes of stretching and strengthening exercises in the first week then try to increase your sessions over time.

Perform low-key and low-impact exercises like moving about and ensure you limit sitting down in front of a computer or a television. Take a walk, use the stairs, ride a bike, or do stretches between breaks at your work place to improve blood flow and boost your energy. Pilates and tai chi are also good exercises when suffering from chronic fatigue. You don't have to do all of these in the first week; just do the ones you can.

Avoid heavy weight lifting, intense aerobic, running sprints, and other high intensity exercises, which can make your muscles sore and worsen fatigue.

Yoga is also an effective remedy for CFS. Let's take a quick look at yoga as a remedy for chronic fatigue.

(I) Yoga

Yoga exercises affect the mind, body, energy, and emotions. It's an effective fatigue treatment as it combines rest, movement, and stress reduction while fostering life force energy and initiating restoration. In the process, it addresses the emotional, physical, and energetic fatigue causes, and promotes and aids in self-inquiry and self-observation in order to understand the triggers of tension.

The following yoga poses will provide rest, improve blood oxygen and nutrient circulations hence increase your energy and reduce general fatigue. Ensure to keep breathing in and out during the entire exercise. Do the following yoga poses throughout the first week-if you don't get time to do all of them in the first week, you can do them later in the month. Well, this doesn't mean you should do them in week 1 only; you should ensure to repeat them every single week throughout the month and continue doing them even after the program ends. In simple terms, you should make them part of your exercise regime if you want to emerge successful in your quest to dealing with chronic fatigue successfully.

Try to do any or all the yoga poses below:

Legs up the wall pose

1. Place a mat or blanket on the ground 5 to 6 inches away from the wall. In case you are stiffer, place support lower and further away from the wall and if you are more flexible, place it closer to the wall and higher. Also, move closer to the wall if you are short and further if you are tall.

2. Sit facing sideways on the right end of your support and place your right side

on the wall. Breathe in deeply and make a single smooth movement; put your legs up the wall and slowly lower your shoulders and head down to the ground then exhale. Your sitting bones should touch the space between your support and the wall.

3.   Bend your knees and raise your pelvis from the support with your feet pressing against the wall. Tuck in your support to raise it higher then slowly drop your pelvis back on it.

4.   Raise and release your skull base further from the back of your neck and relax your throat. Move your stratum towards your chin. If the cervical spine feels flat, take a roll of a material and place under your neck. Relax your shoulders and put your arms and hands to your sides with palms up.

5.   Hold your legs relatively enough up against the wall. Release your belly weight and the thighbones into your torso towards the rear side of your

pelvic. Relax your eyes and look down and deep into your heart. Hold this pose for 5 to 15 minutes.

Bridge Pose

1. Place your back flat on the floor and to protect your neck put something like a blanket under your shoulders.

2. Bend your knees and place your feet on the ground very close to your sitting bones. Press your feet and arms into the floor and raise your tailbone up towards the pubis.

3. Lift the butt while firming it off the ground. Keep your inner feet and thighs parallel. Extend your arms and hold your hands below the pelvis to keep your weight on your shoulders. Raise your buttocks parallel to the ground keeping your knees pressed forward away from the hips and directly over your heels. Extend the

tailbone and position it behind your knees.

4. Raise your pelvis in the direction of your navel. Pull your chin away from the sternum and press down the shoulder blades against the back. Push the sternum towards your chin. Open up your shoulders, press down your outer arms, and try to lift off the ground at the neck base into the torso. Hold the pose for 10-30 seconds then release while breathing out and placing the spine gently down to the ground.

Lion Pose

1. Start by kneeling on the ground and placing the right ankle front below the left ankle back. Your feet will point towards the sides.

2. Sit back placing your perineum on top of the right heel.

3. Put your palms (with fingers spread out) on your knees and press them down.

4. Inhale deeply through the nose and at the same time, open your mouth widely and put out your tongue and bend the tip down towards your chin and open out your and gaze them on the tip of your nose. Exhale slowly using the front throat muscles over your throat back then through your mouth producing a 'ha' sound.

5. Produce a roar two to three times then switch the cross to the other ankle and repeat the steps.

As you come to the end of the week, it is important that you must have followed the suggestions above to increase your chances of success. Exercise and diet should be done hand in hand since these will ultimately determine your levels of energy; if you take too much food and gain weight or take the wrong foods (those that heighten chronic fatigue), you are likely to be sluggish and lack energy, which is a characteristic of chronic fatigue syndrome.

Everything you do in week one will be repeated in week two and the subsequent weeks throughout the program so don't just stop following the stuff you've learnt in week 1 when week 2 comes. Let's now move on to week 2.

Week 2: Relax And Be Happy

Patience is a very important virtue when it comes to these programs. I believe by the end of the first week, you have felt some improvements in your body. Let's now move on swiftly and look at what we are going to do in week two:

Start Getting Enough Sleep

Good sleep reenergizes you and prevents energy exhaustion because of keeping you awake, which requires an extra amount of energy. Lack of enough quality sleep is a major cause of chronic fatigue because it prevents your body from resting properly and interferes with the overall performance of your body organs. Your busy life and stresses could interfere with your sleeping patterns causing you to sleep less than is recommended.

An adult requires 7-9 hours of sleep every night to ensure the body functions properly. Also, try to make an effort of going to bed and waking up around the same time to establish a stable sleep pattern. If you sleep at 11pm and wake up at 6pm over the weekday, try to do so even during the weekend. Establishing a sleep cycle is very important in helping you get the kind of rest you want.

If you find yourself always yawning and tired when not hungry or bored, it's a sign that your system needs to shut down due to poor sleeping habits. You can take an afternoon nap to regain wakefulness, increase performance, and boost your energy. Avoid napping for more than 30 minutes during the day to avoid nighttime sleeping troubles.

Taking too much caffeine, especially in the evening can cause you to have insomnia so limit use and especially avoid taking it after dinner or before bedtime. When you get to bed don't start thinking of your problems; you should relax and let your mind switch off naturally. Some of the sleeping techniques you can use include; thinking of a serene place like the ocean or waterfalls, listening to your breath, or repeating a phrase or mantra in silence.

Using your cell phone in bed is a habit that takes away your valuable sleep so switch it off or mute to avoid sleep disruptions. Avoid using sleeping pills since they are only superficial solutions and do not address the root cause of your sleeping problems; they could also create a dependency of some sort.

Relaxation And Stress Relief Techniques

If you notice that you are having a hard time getting enough sleep, it is very probable that you are suffering from stress and other psychological problems. Meditation and other relaxation techniques can help with this. Let's take a quick look at these and how to go about it:

(m) Meditation

Meditation is a practice that enhances deep spiritual connections, freedom from the material world struggles and inner peace. It allows you to take a break from your stress and worries enhancing relaxation and peace. Find time to meditate daily no matter how busy you are and choose a quiet place. Discipline is required to enable you stay motionless and block all thoughts, feelings and stimulants from interfering with the calm state of your body and mind. Let thoughts flow in and out effortlessly without trying so hard to push them away, just keep your focus. Start with 5-10 minutes then increase the duration gradually as you become better at it. The benefits of meditation include enhancing sleep, reducing stress and increasing energy among other benefits. This makes it effective in eliminating some of the causes of fatigue and reducing on symptoms.

Meditation is an activity you can practice in your house unless you feel the need to take a class as a beginner.

Here are some simple techniques that will help you start meditation. These will help you connect with your inner self, release body and mind tension, and revitalize your body. Do them in the morning and, or late afternoon. As you do the routines in week two, it is important to note that these don't necessarily need to be done in week 2 only; you have to do them in the other weeks (try to create time for them) for you to derive the much needed success in conquering your chronic fatigue problems. So, what meditation techniques should you try to do this week?

Here are a few of them:

(n) Relaxation Meditation Technique

1. Sit on a comfortable mat or chair, cross your legs inward. Sit straight and ensure your spine is straight, chest open and shoulders relaxed. With the palms facing up, rest your hands on your lap or knees. Relax the jaw, face, and belly. Place your tongue on the roof of your mouth, right behind your front teeth. Close your eyes slightly.

2.   Breathe smoothly, slowly and deeply in and out through your nose. Inhale starting from the belly and then rise your breath up into your chest then exhale through your mouth. As you slowly deepen your breath, release all thoughts and distractions and let your mind focus on your breath. Focus deep within the core of your body to find a still, quiet, and peaceful place.

•

3.   Continue to breathe in and out deeply and fill your awareness into this centre. Feel your awareness and breath nourishing this place of inner peace, as it gradually starts to grow and spread outwards. Feel your whole being filled by the expansion of this place of inner peace. Feel your body being entirely saturated by this inner peace as it's released outwards into the world.

(o) Meditation To Increase Energy

1. Lie flat on your bed or sit up straight on a chair in a comfortable posture.

2. Simply move into meditation without trying so hard to push away arising matters. Let yourself go into an attitude of kindness and curiosity
    •

3. Listen to the sound and the sensations of your rhythmic breaths. Just breathe in and out freely and as you breathe in, imagine that you are breathing in fresh, nourishing, and energizing air into your body. Feel the nutritious oxygen enter your entire body. Breathe out imagining that your body is getting rid of all the toxins and let go of any troubling matters, negative emotions and thoughts.

4. Feel more revitalized and elevated with every breath you take. Imagine that you are a jar full of energy interchanging with the energy that surrounds you. Feel this exchange of

energy with every breath you take. Sense the give and take process happening.

•

5.   Bring yourself back to awareness of your breathing. Breathe in and out with a caring, acceptance, and empathetic spirit.

6. As you finish your meditation, be aware of your shift into a regular, alert state.

As you go about your daily activities, think of this energy exchange that surrounds you.

Manage Your Stress

Stress interferes with how your body functions. For instance, when you are stressed, a hormone known as cortisol is usually released and this hormone is usually responsible for the "flight or fight" response, whereby, your body tries to reduce the amount of energy used for various functions so that you have adequate energy to fight or flee, when you are actually in no threat. Consistent high levels of cortisol can make you on edge always, making it even hard to have a good night's rest. This can then lead to tiredness and within no time, you will be suffering from chronic fatigue.

While I know it can be hard to avoid stress, what you can do is find ways of managing the stress. For instance, if you have a schedule that makes you stressed all the time, start by making your schedule flexible and creating simple, measurable, attainable, realistic, and time bound goals. Also, limit on television and news, as most news are full of horrific or disturbing stories which are so much dramatized that they leave you feeling like you actually witnessed the occurrence hence shocking your system and raising your stress level. Other ways of avoiding stress as well as dealing with stress include:

*When listening to music, ensure to keep the volume on your device low enough to hear without straining your ears to avoid thought disruptions, which can bring stress to an otherwise relaxing activity.

*Having a personal journal where you note down what makes you unhappy or stressed and all things that make you happy, calm, and lift your moods and make you feel much better. Although everyone is different, it has been established that noting down what you experience and enjoy can help you adjust your priorities and focus on more crucial things that enrich your life. Additionally, noting down what may not make you happy is a way of dealing with any frustration and pent up anger.

*Doing one thing at a time and making sure you rest in between or after your scheduled activities to enable the body to cool down, regain energy and avoid burnouts.

(p) Try Cognitive Behavioral Therapy

This type of therapy is known for working wonders and it is a perfect activity for a chronic fatigued patient. It mainly helps you deal with chronic fatigue syndrome by teaching you how to change the way you think and behave. It is said that you are what you think and this goes on to show you how important your mind is and how it plays a big role in your life.

Chronic fatigue syndrome has very many symptoms and this therapy mostly uses different methods to deal with different symptoms. Since everyone requires a tailor made cognitive behavioral therapy, you need to know the exact symptom that you have so that your therapist can be of use to you.

Cognitive behavioral therapy reduces the severity of your symptoms and the suffering that comes with CFS. This therapy works by breaking down your huge problems and put them in small categories where it is easy to solve them. It also breaks down the negative interconnected thoughts, feelings, actions, and physical sensations that people have. This process is normally carried out by a therapist who is well trained in the field of chronic fatigue syndrome. The therapy helps you to:

*Increase your control senses so that you can avoid your symptoms controlling you.

*Accept your diagnosis

*Deal with challenging feelings that can stand in the way of your symptoms improving.

*This process is used to as a treatment for other long-term conditions like cancer but this does not mean that CFS is a psychological condition.

Tip: You should also try to get a massage during this week to help you with relaxation and to help you to manage chronic fatigue with greater ease.

Week 3: Supplementation and Detox Week

By now, you have probably started noticing patterns of things, tendencies, and symptoms of CFS that seem to just not go away. This is why you should ensure to write down what it is you notice as you go on with the program to ensure you can easily spot any patterns.

Supplements offer a great alternative if your diet is not well balanced. Consider taking quality vitamin and mineral supplements after consulting with a homeopathic doctor or nutritionist. So, what is it you should be taking? Let's learn that next:

What Vitamins and Minerals To Take

Your diet should have sufficient amounts of essential minerals and vitamins, which will promote your body energy hence ending fatigue. Deficiency in these important elements causes fatigue among other conditions. Here are the most important minerals and vitamins that you should have in your diet if your symptoms are not going away.

Thiamin (vitamin B1)

Thiamin is necessary for carbohydrate metabolism, and a high dietary intake of carbohydrates necessitates a higher intake of thiamine. Thiamine content in food is reduced by moist heat, Sulphites and alkalis like baking soda. The suitable daily intake of this vitamin if you are experiencing chronic fatigue is 2 to 10mg daily of thiamine. Foods high in thiamine include oats, sunflower, barley, Lima greens, dried peas, green peas, and black beans.

Riboflavin (vitamin B2)

Riboflavin aids in energy production, mitochondrial function, detox, cell protection, lipid metabolism, and chemical detoxification processes. It also aids folic acid pyridoxine, vitamin K, and niacin metabolism.

Exercise increases the need for riboflavin. Alcohol, alkalis, and caffeine interfere with riboflavin. If chronically fatigued, you should take about 2 to 10 mg daily. Soybean spinach, tempeh, greens, yoghurt, eggs, and mushrooms are some of the foods containing vitamin B2.

Niacin and niacinamide (vitamin B3)

Niacin highly promotes energy production from fats and carbohydrates, mitochondrial function, and maintains blood lipid levels.

If you have chronic fatigue, you should take around 30 to 100 mg daily. To avoid liver toxicity, don't take niacin in higher doses.

Pantothenic acid (vitamin B5)

Pantothenic acid aids in protein and carbohydrate metabolism and helps in stress management. You need to take 10 to 50 mg daily. Mushrooms, avocado, lentils, chicken, and broccoli are some great sources.

Pyridoxine (vitamin B6)

Pyridoxine helps in protein metabolism hence reducing fatigue. If chronically fatigued, take about 10 to 25 mg daily. Sweet potato, fish, sunflower, spinach, and bananas are some of its sources.

Cobalamin (vitamin B12)

Cobalamin promotes body oxygenation process and its deficiency causes fatigue. If chronically fatigued, take about 30 to 100 micrograms daily. Fish, beef, and yogurt are good sources.

Biotin

Biotin aids in carbohydrate, protein, and fatty acid metabolism. It also helps balance energy levels and maintain skin, hair and nail health. If chronically fatigued, you are advised to take approximately 100 to 300 micrograms daily.

Vitamin C

Vitamin C protects your body's energy

producing cells and systems. Frequent intake is necessary because it's passed out easily by your body. If chronically fatigued, take about 500 to 1000 mg daily. Strawberry, papaya, Brussels sprouts, pineapple, oranges, bell pepper, and cantaloupe are some of the great sources.

Vitamin E

Vitamin E is an antioxidant and aids in protecting fatty acids, blood cells, and fats circulating in the blood. If chronically fatigued, take about 400 to 600 IU daily. Some of its great sources include almonds, asparagus, beet greens, peanut, avocado, sunflower, and spinach.

Magnesium

Magnesium promotes mitochondrial function, muscular function, fat, protein, and carbohydrate metabolism. If chronically fatigued, take about 400 to 600 mg daily. Sesame seeds, quinoa, soybeans, cashew and navy beans are some great sources

Iron

Iron promotes blood cell formation and if deficient, you are likely to suffer from fatigue. Therefore, aim to take 10 mg daily. Some of its great sources include lentils, garbanzo beans, Lima seeds, kidney beans, olives, and Swiss chard.

Zinc

Zinc promotes carbohydrate and hormone metabolism, cell protection and growth, and immune function. The thing about zinc is that its absorption decreases with age. If chronically fatigued, take 15 to 30 mg daily. Some great sources are; lamb, shrimp, beef, turkey, and pumpkin seeds.

Chromium

Chromium is a mineral that promotes carbohydrate and fat metabolism. High intake of sugar decreases this mineral in your body. Its deficiency changes your body's response to simple carbohydrates in your diet and upsets blood sugar and blood lipid levels. If chronically fatigued, take 50 to 200 micrograms daily. Some sources include fruits such as bananas and apples, tomatoes, black pepper, oats, romaine lettuce, and barley

Selenium

Selenium is an antioxidant and if chronically fatigued take about 70 to 200 micrograms daily. Sources include tuna, lamb, turkey, chicken, scallops, and beef.

Iodine

Iodine promotes body detoxification functions. If chronically fatigued, take 100 to 200 micrograms daily. Sea or table salt is a great source

Vanadium

Vanadium is a trace mineral that aids in metabolism of glucose. If chronically fatigued, take about 10 to 50 micrograms daily. Some sources include grains, olive oil, green beans, soy, cabbage, carrots, garlic, and wine.

L-Carnitine

L-carnitine is a compound that is important in body functioning. It transports fatty fuels to mitochondria, removes wastes, and maintains blood lipid and blood sugar levels. Animal foods, vitamins B3, C, and B6 and iron aid in its production. If chronically fatigued, take about 1 to 3 grams daily. Some sources include meat and dairy products.

Coenzyme Q10

Coenzyme Q10 (CoQ10) promotes mitochondrial function and has antioxidant properties. Some of its sources include spinach, fish, meats, beans, and nuts. Your average daily dietary intake is about 2 to 5 mg. If chronically fatigued, take about 50 to 200 mg daily.

By now, your body has started to feel better

and you can't compare it with the weakness that you had before we started this procedure.

Detox

How does toxicity affect your health? Let me use a simple method to explain; your body is like a glass of water in that it takes in toxins and the more it takes, the more the glass gets filled up. So finally, the glass ends up overflowing with toxins because it is full and that's where diseases start showing up in your life. Although the body can naturally detox itself, it is likely to be overwhelmed by such things like:

*Heavy metals like lead and mercury, pesticides, residues and petrochemicals

*Some of the unhealthy foods that we eat

*Food allergies, toxins from moles and environmental allergies

*Stress that triggers inefficiencies in our body's ability to detox

*Medication can be another form of toxic.

*You can't avoid using medication but overmedication can bring more harm than good.

*Lastly, we all have internal toxics such as fungus, yeast, bacteria, hormonal and metabolic toxins that are inside our gut.

Some people are good in dealing with toxins in their bodies while others like chronic fatigue syndrome patients are not. That's why you should learn how to use the method that I am going to discuss to put an end to your chronic fatigue problem.

How to detox

NOTE: The purpose of this week's detox is to push your body to detox itself naturally without having to go to extreme lengths with the detox like going on a green smoothie fast or taking raw food. Before you get started, you need to take note of some 5 important guidelines:

*Identify the toxin and get rid of it

*Fix your source of toxic load, which is your gut

*Let your blood and lymphatic circulation do their job

*Ensure you get your liver and detox system working

*Make sure you detox your mind, heart and spirit.

Let me now make it more practical for you in the following steps that you can easily follow to detox your body:

*Make sure you drink plenty of clean water in a day preferably eight to ten glasses.

*If you can't keep your bowels moving once or twice in a day then you need to help yourself by taking two tablespoons of ground flax seeds or taking extra magnesium capsules which are in the form of magnesium citrate.

*You should include organic produce and animal products like, meat and eggs in your diet in order to eliminate the toxins that we normally get from other foods.

*Make sure you eat eight to ten servings of fruits and vegetables every day. You should include foods such as vegetables, kales, sprouts, Brussels, cabbage, broccoli, collards, garlic and onion, which help you to increase the levels of sulfur in your body and help in detoxification.

*You should avoid stimulants, sedatives and drugs such as nicotine and caffeine because they just fill your body with toxins.

*Involve yourself in exercises five days a week where you focus on conditioning your cardiovascular system, stretching exercises, and strengthening exercises.

*Get rid of foods that bring more harm than

good like the menace of white flour and white sugar. These types of foodstuffs should be taken in low quantities because they end up being toxic to your body.

*Find some methods, which can make you sweat profusely like three times a week: a good example is jogging, steam, using a sauna or having a detox bath.

*Take foods rich in high quality minerals and multivitamins like fruits and vegetables.

*Lastly, you should make sure you get your nervous system in a state of calm, rest and in a relaxation mode. Make sure you have a routine of relaxing deeply every day.

The steps that we have outlined above will help you control the amount of toxicity in your body, maximize the detoxification of your body, and help you to eliminate the stored toxins in your body. You should try and detox every day this week. This will go a long way towards fighting chronic fatigue.

But if you feel you are up to it, you can go on a 3 day green smoothie cleanse. In this case, all you have to do is to take smoothies exclusively for a few days. So, how do you do the cleanse? Here is a green smoothie recipe that will help you with detoxification:

Ingredients

1 tablespoon of fresh organic lemon juice
1 banana
1 pear, cored and chopped
1 apple, cored and chopped
1 ½ cups of chopped celery
6 cups of chopped romaine lettuce
7 cups of chopped spinach
2 cups of cold and filtered water

Directions

Blend all ingredients until smooth.

NOTE: Ensure to take dark green veggies like bok choy, beet greens, arugula, lettuce, kale, dandelion greens, collard greens, Swiss chard, carrot top leaves, radish tops, spinach, watercress, turnip greens, spring greens etc. You can add in a few fruits to taste but if you still feel it is not as sweet, add some sweeteners like stevia.

(q) Pacing

This process involves you balancing your activity time with your resting time. Most CFS patients think that when they push themselves to the limit they accomplish more and heal faster. However, when you overdo an activity beyond your limits, you are only hurting yourself. You are likely to overcome chronic fatigue when you balance your activities with some rest, then maybe later on you can gradually increase your periods of activities as you do the same for the resting periods.

This method is the difference between progress and stagnation in the journey towards fighting CFS. You should sit down every day and try to balance the amount of activity you are planning to do with the amount of resting time that you will give yourself. Create an environment that promotes smooth flow of activities and your week three will be as easy as a Sunday morning.

Week 4: Time To Get More Hands On

It's not how you start but how you finish. That is the thought that comes into my head as we take on our last week where we will say goodbye to all our CFS problematic symptoms. To get through the fourth week, it is important that I point out that you will be introducing new treatments to help you relax and combat chronic fatigue with a lot of ease. We will start with essential oils:

Introduce Essential Oils

Essential oils are liquid plant extracts and using them as a treatment therapy cures or prevents many conditions including fatigue, stress and sleep problems.

Applying essential oils requires you to use carrier oils, which include coconut oil, almond oil, olive oil, grape seed oil and canola oil or a vegetable oil. This dilutes essential oils to prevent skin irritation caused by using pure ones directly on the skin. Test on the inside part of your upper arm section before use to see whether you are sensitive to a particular essential oil. So what essential oils should you use this week? We will learn all that next:

Lemon Balm

Lemon Balm essential oil has been used in many places to relieve stress and anxiety, which are some of the causes of fatigue. In order to use, mix 2 drops of lemon balm with 1 drop of a vegetable oil then rub into your hands, and breathe in the aroma to relax your mind and body.

Rosemary

Rosemary essential oil contains a chemical called 1.8 cineole, which increases the cerebral blood flow that helps reduce fatigue.

To use rosemary essential oil, take a ball of cotton and put a drop of rosemary essential oil on it then inhale once through each nostril.

Alternatively, using rosemary essential oil you can create a personal nasal inhaler. This enables you to carry your inhaler wherever you go. The nasal inhalers last for two to three months. Add 2 to 3 drops mixed with a shower gel to a bathing towel and massage it to the body. Use it once a day for 30-90 days for best results.

Aromatherapy for energy recipe

Try the recipe below to help you fight off the symptoms that come with chronic fatigue:

Ingredients

1 drop of cinnamon leaf oil
2 drops of eucalyptus oil
2 ounces of vegetable oil
8 drops of lemon oil
2 drops of peppermint oil
1 drop of cardamom oil (optional)

Instructions

Mix all the ingredients in a jar then put in a

dark bottle. For your body bath, add 2 teaspoons of the essential oil blend and for a footbath, add 1 teaspoon to the water. You can make a diffuser without the vegetable oil or an air spray using 2 ounces of water. Use the mixture as often as you desire.

Introduce Herbs For Fatigue

Herbs have been used for centuries in the treatment of various conditions including fatigue. Here are some few herbs you can incorporate in your fight against fatigue.

Note: Ensure to consult with a specialist before ingesting the herbs.

Maca root

Maca is a root that can be used to ease fatigue symptoms and enhance blood flow. You can make liquid extracts and root powder or eat the whole raw root sliced, boiled cooked, or baked. Take a teaspoon of the powder and mix in a cup of water or tea. You can also sprinkle it on food or take it as a capsule.

Licorice Tonic for Fatigue

Licorice herb helps rebuild impaired adrenals and lessens your craving for caffeine and sugars hence eliminates energy crash. The glycyrrhizin compound in licorice root improves on the cortisol hormone and enhances energy hence eases fatigue.

Ingredients

1 stick licorice root, medium, broken pieces
4-inch fresh ginger, medium, sliced
1 tablespoon reishi root, chopped
½ teaspoon powdered spice mix (cloves, cardamom, and sweet cinnamon)

Instructions

Bring 2 liters of water to boil, over low heat, and then simmer for 10 minutes. There is no need to strain because the herbs settle at the bottom of the pot. Take a glass and pour the tea then keep the rest in a jug in the refrigerator. Take once daily, in the morning for two or three weeks and rest one week in between.

Conclusion

Thank you again for downloading this book!
I hope this book was able to help you to know how to get rid of chronic fatigue.

Thank you again for downloading this book!

I hope this book was able to help you to know how to get rid of chronic fatigue.

The next step is to try the 30-day challenge where you incorporate the strategies outlined in this book in order to overcome your fatigue.

CPSIA information can be obtained at www.ICGtesting.com
Printed in the USA
LVOW04s0104190915

454879LV00040B/1010/P